I0414672

SO YOU HAD A HEART ATTACK SUCK IT UP BUTTERCUP

DAVID SEABOLT

SO YOU HAD A HEART ATTACK SUCK IT UP BUTTERCUP

DEDICATION

This book is dedicated to my wife, children, and grandchildren as an apology for having scared them so terribly. My ignorance and stubbornness caused all my loved ones unnecessary pain and fear and I hope to help someone else, maybe you the reader, to reclaim your life after the, "Big One".

FOREWORD

Some people may assume that as an author on the subject of heart attacks that I have some fancy credentials or at least letters behind my name to prove my authority in matters relative to such things. Nope, not here. My authority on the subject extends as far as and is completely limited to my personal experiences before, during, and after my, "event". We've all heard the phrase, Experience is the best teacher, my experience is all I'm offering here. Legal disclosures to follow but primarily I do not wish to cause anyone harm and so don't be stupid. If my experiences are in conflict with yours, don't ignore your medical, emotional, and/or spiritual advisors on my account. Because Dave said won't help you at the pearly gates!

I've started this literary journey with my heart attack and ended it with where I am relative to all things considered relevant to my heart attack and my current day to day survival. Within the separate chapters however you will see me bounce around a little in my efforts to reinforce specific points of interest. I will surely sound like a broken record because you will read many times that I'm not a health care professional. This is because I wish for you to gain benefits from this work and not provide you with justifications for poor life choices. Don't blame me or this book. Stand on your own two feet and make **YOUR** life worth having and sharing! Buttercup!

CONTENTS

1 THE EVENT

Well here we go folks. Every heart attack experience is different and in my case several factors were certainly in my favor. My attack occurred at work where I had a direct connection to emergency response agencies and from point of self-diagnosis to having an ambulance at my location was about fifteen minutes. The ride was about twenty minutes and the stent was placed within approximately an hour after I decided that I must be having a heart attack.

Without giving away too much I hope, my job involves playing on the freeway. Just like my momma told me to do. I work on vehicles, sometimes in live travel lanes, to keep traffic moving as smoothly as possible. A little stressful at times? Yes, for sure but I've worked in some wild environments before. I usually came out of those experiences intact so playing on the freeway at the age of fifty-one was no big deal to me. My job, most of the time, is driving around in big circles and listening to music while avoiding poor driving behaviors with a smile and a wave. Actually, my boss told me that I'm not allowed to wave anymore…

It was a warm day in May and I had just changed a flat tire caused during a crash, thus allowing the vehicle to leave the freeway. I put my tools away and climbed into the driver's seat, immediately turning up the A/C. Boy was I sweating! It was about eighty degrees so I didn't worry too much about the mild head rush I was feeling as the A/C began to take effect. No big deal, just another day at the office. I completed my paperwork and pulled away from the scene and now I was really feeling the cold sweat and rush that I thought was coming from the effects of good A/C. Yeah, I was wrong. I continued driving for about five minutes waiting for these feelings to pass and began drinking more water. I thought maybe I was just a little dehydrated; I'd been there and back before. Again, no big deal, right? Wrong! I began losing vision and focus in a way I had never done before. This was serious and I was now a rolling grenade with the pin pulled!

My heartfelt, self-righteous concern for the safety and welfare of the general motoring public finally overcame my pride and confidence so I pulled over in the safest location I could immediately find. Fortunately I had a radio, remember that direct line to emergency response? I requested medical assistance to my location. The dispatcher initially responded in the affirmative without much thought. About three minutes later the dispatcher called me back and asked who I needed medical attention for since I had not logged a stop with another vehicle. When I told them it was for me personally they expedited the call and within about two minutes I had two state troopers on scene with me! It's nice to have connections.

Ever the sarcastic I enjoy the dark humor residing in many frightening situations. So, when the ambulance arrived and the paramedics came to me and asked what the issue was I said that I THOUGHT that I might be having a heart attack but I wasn't sure and it sure would be embarrassing if it wasn't the case. Yes, I am the one that laughs at inappropriate circumstances at the wrong time. Apparently I am not alone in my shortcoming because after the paramedic hooked me up to the monitors she said, "Congratulations, you're having a heart attack". I tried to laugh, by the way that's not an easy thing to do in those circumstances. Did you try to laugh when the air was knocked out of you and everything was closing in on you? Still I prefer humor and appreciated the paramedic's humor very much. In fact I can never express to all persons that responded to my situation how very much I appreciate their time, knowledge, commitment, and yes of course their humor as they saved my life! Enough gooey stuff for now.

Before I knew it I was at the emergency entrance at the hospital and being rushed to the, "Cath Lab". More of my heroes were waiting for me in the lab as if they had been waiting for me all day. The reality was that they, the lab staff, were in the parking lot having ended their shift and were headed home when they were called back to the lab for me. I love great timing! Experiences may vary. A close friend of mine had to wait several hours from his time of admission to the emergency ward before stents were placed and he's fine, kinda. Physically and mentally the wait had no discernable impact on my friend but I'm told that my event certainly would not have allowed for that time-table.

With my legal disclosure in full effect here, I am reminded of part of my ride to the hospital that I feel needs to be highlighted. I bring this up because it will bear greatly both in my concern for anyone having a heart attack as well as the humor of subsequent events that occurred in the Cath Lab. The discourse between the young paramedic lady and I went something like this. She asked if I would be willing to receive some nitroglycerin to help expand my blood vessels. She went on to say that sometimes people will refuse medications for religious and other beliefs. My response and I hope yours as well if you ever find yourself in a similar situation was an emphatic, "Yes I'll take it, whatever keeps me breathing"! Of course if you're reading this because you experienced the great event, congratulations, you made the right decisions!

Anyway, back at the Cath Lab the staff transferred me from my gurney to the operating table and started removing clothes and hooking me up to all kinds of equipment. Was my underwear clean? I wondered. Damn I'm fat and ugly! In the moment my vanity showed up and I had to send it away. The staff was amazing and the doctor effective. After examination the doctor and staff agreed that I needed a stent placed in one of my coronary arteries as a result of a total occlusion. Basically I had a clot that had completely stopped blood flow to one of my heart chambers.

The next point of humor for me was when the staff told me the doctor was going to go through my wrist to install the stent but in case of complications they would prep me for alternative access at my groin! As they unceremoniously pulled my pants and underwear down I couldn't help thinking that I wouldn't be a very impressive specimen to the female staff. When they went at me with a disposable razor I remembered that I wanted to live even though I was embarrassed and hopefully I wouldn't see these ladies again anyway! Everyone was so professional and soon I was half shaved, pants at my ankles and the doctor ready to try at my wrist. The white hot sensation I felt when he cut open my wrist was surprising and scary as hell. Was I going to bleed out? I didn't know that my blood was so hot! A personal note to medical professionals, please prepare your patients for that experience. I was already freaking out, not able to breathe, and feeling like the lights were going out.

When the stent was placed and the artery back open for business, WOW! Instant relief as my heart started pumping blood again! I didn't care about being an impressive specimen or embarrassed, I was going to live! Finally someone covered me with a blanket, for my dignity or their disinterest I did not know which, nor did I care. Everyone was smiling and I felt their relief and sense of pride knowing they had saved my life. For a few moments we were all allies in a successful campaign, victorious friends!

The moment quickly passed as the doctor reassured me that I would make it and the staff started tidying up the lab. One of the nurses entered the room with a look of total disbelief and asked me if all those people out there were for me. Oh damn, the only communication I'd had with my wife was a text telling her that I loved her before the ambulance arrived and the lab staff had taken my phone some time before stripping me. "I don't know; who's out there?" I said. "Your wife and a bunch of other people", She responded. "The waiting room is overflowing. I don't think we've ever had so many here for one person before. You must be very loved." She continued with a grin. By the way, YES I AM!

Before they let me see anyone they showed me the procedure on a monitor that gave me the visual of my blocked artery and the restart of the blood flow when the stent was opened. At that moment my wife entered the room as a lab tech and I were laughing about the humor we had observed during the procedure. Her look of fear and tears of stress at thinking she might have lost me were suddenly gone and anger and frustration immediately replaced them. "Here I'm worried sick that you're dying and I come in to see you and a nurse laughing and joking like nothing happened? I should hit you for doing this to me!" She broke into tears and we held hands as I cried with her.

Lucky to live in these times, I thought. No open heart procedures or worse no medical interventions available in years before could have meant my certain death. After my new cardiologist visited with me in my hospital room I learned just how important time was but I'll get into that later in the book.

After the blur of consoling my wife and children with hand grips, kisses, and tears. After telling them it was just a little thing, no big deal, trying to believe it as I said it. I was taken to ICCU and set up in a room. The hospital staff were fantastic if maybe, as I felt, a bit over cautious. Bed pans and call buttons were the primary topics, no trying to get up or turning around in the bed. Two hours ago I was changing tires on the freeway and now I can't get up on my own to take a leak? Really? I wanted to go home. After all my heart was working fine and I felt like Superman after having just survived this crazy scary near death experience!

A quick fast forward here, I later learned that my event was referred to as a STEMI. A STEMI for those new to heart attacks is an occasion when one or more arteries suddenly become totally blocked. The result if not treated quickly is major heart muscle damage. This damage cannot be repaired ever. Remember that in my case I had the stent within one to two hours? Because of that I came away with only a bruised heart. If you've never had a heart attack please remember that time is not your friend, do NOT mess with it! I know people that now may deal with the side effects of beta blocker medications for the rest of their lives because they were not treated in a timely manner. Believe me, while it's good to be alive, it's better if you don't hesitate or allow medical institutions to dally. First and foremost this is YOUR life!

In the hospital I learned that I was indeed far more fortunate than most, again, because of how quickly I had been treated. When I continued to down-play the severity of my experience for my wife's benefit one of the nurses checking my vitals at the time raised her brow and exposed my lie. She informed my wife that this had not been anywhere near a mild heart attack; so much for softening the blow. The rest of my stay included a move to a semi-private room at about three AM on the day I would leave. By the way, if this ever happens to you I highly recommend the bedsore check be provided by two young and pretty nurses! That was certainly a highlight!

One last thing that I did not know before my event is the reason they will not let you out until after the third day at the eaarliest. When you experience a heart attack it wreaks havoc on your heart's electrical system and cause sudden cardiac arrest. The explanation given to me by a nurse was that after the heart endures the trauma associated with a heart attack the electrical system may sometimes reset itself in a violent way. If I was not under observation and at home when the reset occurred I could die. Suddenly I wasn't so pissy about the three night stay! My reset happened on the second night, about twelve irregular heartbeats and everything returned to normal. I didn't even know until a nurse came in and checked my monitor after the alarm went off. I am indeed a fortunate man!

As an aside, my eighty-seven year old grandfather died from sudden cardiac arrest the year following my event. The tough old boy had at least three cardiac arrests in the hospital after his heart attack and just couldn't fight it anymore. Let them keep you for as long as they need to. The bill is not the most important priority!

2 THE PROGNOSIS

For those of you just joining our program, I just experienced a heart attack and now I'm in the hospital in the ICCU. My event was a STEMI, which occurred when a blood clot completely plugged an artery. This resulted in my heart desperately trying to pump a fluid currently not forthcoming. Because I received timely medical attention I was in extremely good shape, all things considered.

During my three day vacation I had opportunity to speak with nurses, doctors, friends, and family. Every medical professional was amazed at my condition and every lay-person had shared experiences or provided guidance for me based on their knowledge. The professionals pushed their recommendations per currently accepted medical information. All in all I was being overwhelmed with well-intended advice while still dealing with my major life altering experience. I also spent a bit of time on the internet researching survival and lifestyle strategies on my own as well. If you had a similar experience after your event I thought you'd like to know that you weren't the only one my friend!

My prognosis was explained in detail by the lady doctor that discharged me and I'll get into that conversation momentarily because I wish to describe a few of my experiences that I can only describe as well intended prognoses from others but some of it I found to be a little misguided.

My son was understandably shaken by the possibility that he'd almost lost his father and he did his best to educate me on the lifestyle choices he believed I needed to make. You can't drink coffee or smoke anymore. You have to find easier work. You need to settle down and take it easy now dad. He'd researched online and firmly believed these things to be true. Now I don't dispute that not smoking and reducing stress were logical considerations but no more coffee and find easier work? I ain't no pansy! I got things to do, I'm not ready to lay down just yet!

Luckily I had checked a few things out myself. Despite all information to the contrary no clinical studies have definitively linked caffeine to heart attacks. Furthermore there are several studies that have concluded that significant coffee drinking, say more than two eight ounce cups per day, may actually have several health benefits. As one friend said after my heart attack, "The coffee probably saved your life."

My well-meaning son and the rest of my family now have to accept that I won't be around forever and understandably they only want me to make better choices so as to stick around longer. If you're a father you need to understand how hard it is for your family to accept that you are no longer ten foot tall and bullet proof. Please be kind to your friends and family as they begin this new part of <u>their</u> life's journey. Accept their concern and panic with a comforting smile and hug. Let them know you understand their fears and let it slide until you can have a less stressful environment for them to be in. I absolutely hate hospitals because people die there!

The hospital sent a dietary consultant to my room to discuss what changes I should consider in my diet. These changes were presented as things I would absolutely need to accommodate if I cared about myself and my family. Really?! I could join a group of heart attack survivors for support, not my style. I could go online to receive dietary guidance and support from professionals, yeah, no. I could be put in touch with religious support, not. The bottom line to the guidance is to eat only lean, white meats, fish, salad, no added salt, you probably know, the standards based on currently stated professional beliefs. Can you tell I'm not a fan? More on that subject in the diet section.

Now the lady doctor that discharged me probably had a few conversations about life after a heart attack before meeting with my wife and I. She was humorous, concise, and even compassionate. Not compassionate to me, my wife! Yes. Me? Not so much. Just kidding. She did a great job explaining what I experienced and how I could proceed towards a longer, healthier life if I wished to do so. To give you a hint at her humor consider her opener, "The days of a carton of cigarettes and two gallons of whiskey a day are done now!" I responded with a grin and looked her in the eye saying, "Those days have been gone for a long time already!" During the conversation she looked at my wife and told her straight out, "No sex for at least a week or two." My wife blushed and looked down saying, "I hadn't really thought about that just yet but why not?" The doctor said to her essentially that men will literally kill themselves to complete the act once it has begun. Well duh!

The doctor explained that my condition was the result of excess cholesterol in the artery breaking loose and plugging the artery. This then caused the blood to clot around the cholesterol thus completely blocking blood flow to one chamber of my heart. As explained by her the best chance I had was to take cholesterol reducing medications, reduce salt intake in order to reduce blood pressure, exercise, reduce fatty foods, eat leaner, greener foods, and lastly reduce stress. Of course I should quit smoking!

According to her the reality of my life is that my genetics are contributory to my circumstances, a recent conversation with my mother, in the hospital, after the attack reinforced this. My mother informed me at that time that her father had died of a heart attack around the age of sixty-five. I later learned that my father's father died around the same age. Both were Southern boys and were also pretty big. I say big in consideration that I stand six foot-two inches tall and at the time of my little party I came in at about two-hundred-sixty pounds. It was all muscle! You do believe me don't you?

So here I am, having to take medications, probably for the rest of my life, and learning that many of my previous behaviors that were normal to me could now greatly shorten my life. Well damn! I'm scared. I never wanted to be on meds and I hate the thought that at any turn I could keel over without warning and just expire. Essentially I was still a grenade with the pin pulled. I could do everything right and still end up with another heart attack and in fact It wasn't if, it was when. Boy I sure could use a drink after hearing that news!

The most meaningful information the discharge doctor gave me was that I should allow myself an adjustment period before making huge life changes. This is because the stress of huge changes alone could immediately put me back in the hospital. Nobody wanted that! Not me, not my family, and certainly not the ICCU staff!

After leaving the hospital I was taking a beta blocker, aspirin, a blood thinner, and a statin to reduce cholesterol in my blood system. The beta blocker messed with my memory and I felt like I was wearing heavy weights when I tried to regain my previous capacities. Apparently I consistently operated on somewhat elevated levels of adrenalin before my event! Don't get me wrong, the event had bruised my heart muscle and I learned that while it wasn't permanent damage it would be at least a year before my heart would be near what it had been. The blood thinner was needed to keep the stent clot free and would be required for at least a year. I would now be taking aspirin for life as well as the statin.

My first office visit at the heart doctor's office was interesting to me. I had been out of the hospital about three months and I get to visit with a nurse? After my vitals and an EKG I get the same information about diet and exercise I received in the hospital along with contact information for a heart attack recovery support program. Did I tell you how interested I was in getting tied up in a support setting before? If not, that's not me I have my support group. Not to say that you shouldn't consider that option if you do need support.

The second visit, three months after that, went without the EKG and I was informed that I was not doing enough to attain the healthy lifestyle necessary for long term survival. Hmm, I had lost over twenty pounds, my blood pressure on meds was about 117/75, my blood sugars were at one-hundred exactly, my bad cholesterol was down to half of the level it was in the hospital, and my good cholesterol had doubled. I'm not doing enough? I was walking in the hills behind my house going about two miles about three days a week, no small feat on beta blockers let me tell you! Not doing enough? Yeah you know what I wanted to say.

The next visit was about thirteen months after the event at which point the doctor told me to eat something! I was at about two-hundred-one pounds at that visit, an almost sixty pound loss since I was in the hospital. My blood pressure was still under 120/80 and my pulse usually came in around the low sixties. My bad cholesterol was at eighty-one and my good cholesterol was up to about thirty-three. The doctor was impressed and told me to keep doing whatever it was I was doing. We ended the blood thinner and the beta blocker, thank goodness! I was feeling pretty good! Not doing enough my ass!

A side note about blood thinners. Please prepare your family, friends, and co-workers. Any scratch will bleed like a severed artery! You won't realize many times when you're bleeding until you feel the blood running down your arm or when somebody else freaks out when they see it. You will scare small children so please let them know that you'll be fine.

3 STRESS

All things considered I believe that stress is the single most important consideration before and after a heart attack. It is typically the underlying factor from which all other factors are inflamed. If you smoke and you are stressed you usually smoke more. If you binge salty, fatty, sugary food you eat large quantities and more often when stressed. If you are trying to remove yourself from your stresses by watching tv, or web surfing, or playing video games instead of walking, running, or lifting you become more sedentary when you are more stressed. None of this even compares in my opinion to the impact of anxiety and worry on your stress levels and therefore the physical impact on your body, diet, and overall sense of well-being!

First and foremost you just went through one of the most stressful and frightening experiences in your life. That by itself is pretty scary. After my attack I really felt my mortality for the first time. This is not to say that I haven't experienced close calls before. I just always felt that my body was an ally and now our alliance is not as solid as I once believed. I learned that I had not been good to my body and now it had rebelled against me. I realize that I thought that my body was so resilient it could easily overcome the hardships I had put it through. You know; smoking, drinking, long and hard work schedules, and such. My body had managed to stay strong and able to meet the challenges I had put in front of it, until it failed.

Now I was afraid to eat too much or the wrong thing. I had to consider not smoking anymore, and not drinking anymore. A whole new lifestyle that maybe I wouldn't like. I think it was George Burns that said in a joke that without women, whiskey, and cigars he wouldn't want to live. My attitude became simply how much can I keep and still live long and well.

Being told that since I had had an event it wasn't if but when the next one would occur and how damaging it would be. That fear alone has been known to end people, don't let it get you too!

In my experiences since my event I learned that by determining how best to manage your typical stress factors and working at them without excuses will be very beneficial to you. You know the ones; My boss is a jerk; My wife doesn't get it; I still gotta work and can't change to a less stressful profession; My favorite is, "Why? I have all kinds of medications to control the effects of my stresses that I didn't have before?" All of these perspectives can validate poor behaviors and could be used as justifications for the next event and maybe should be on your headstone but… If you want to give yourself the best chance at a high quality of life for the longest possible period then you need to give up on excuses and do the work!

Please understand that I'm a child of the sixties/seventies which means I grew up around free love and daring, irresponsible behaviors. I also learned to adopt the tough guy attitude when it came to pain or discomfort, both emotional and physical. No pussy here right? These attitudes, at least in my case and maybe yours too, taught me the best approach was to toughen up and hide my weaknesses. In other words to internalize my troubles or, suck it up buttercup! Of course explosive outbursts and cutting cynicisms were useful venting methods but they never seemed to bring any real sense of calm to me. Now don't get me wrong, I had an effective modus operandi that worked for more than fifty years but after my heart attack I realized that if I wanted to continue breathing I might want to learn new and more effective methods to managing my stress.

So, what new ways did I find? Well, how about we look at the ones I considered and how I moved forward.

Belligerent conflict was one of my first attempts at managing my stress; a slight modification of my previous behaviors. "Don't piss me off or I might have another heart attack!" "You all need to back off and let me relax!" Sound familiar? Denial of personal responsibility was a standard tactic before the event and using it to get my way after the event was no more or less than an extension of previous bad behaviors. You will probably attempt to use previously effective practices to initially reduce your stress and anxiety. Maybe what, "worked", in the past put you where you're at today?

Spiritual awareness was an approach I tried and actually, while I don't expect to become a Shaman, Preacher, or Guru, I found some new ways to at least reframe my perspective. This has helped me to focus more on the true weight of things rather than my inflated sense of self and the circumstances I live in. My personal experience is of course colored by my past experiences in regard to spiritualism and religion. The tree huggers, hippies, Catholics, Protestants, Jews, and Muslims are all large groups of people that believe what they believe and in my experience believe they have it all figured out relative to where they will end up and what constitutes wrong behavior, usually for others and not themselves. Unfortunately my experiences have led me to believe that religions are primarily self-serving and do very little for the soul unless you become blindly fanatic. I'm done preaching here but my point is if you cannot find a way to accept that you are actually quite a miniscule speck of dust riding this spinning speck of dust in a never ending universe then you will spend an inordinate amount of effort trying to overcome what is. If that doesn't increase your stress level then what else could?

Meditation is still a challenging but fairly fruitful behavior for me. To meditate by definition is think deeply or focus one's mind for a period of time, in silence or with the aid of chanting, for religious or spiritual purposes or as a method of relaxation. If you take away the religious and spiritual purposes you are left with a method of relaxation. I use meditation from time to time to focus on the truly necessary things in life, breathing, muscular and emotional tensions, love, and so on. When I remember that without the simple act of breathing nothing else is possible I usually realize that my concerns of the moment probably mean little in the grand scheme of things. Just breathe and consider things from a relaxed angle. It will help even if only a little.

Alone time has some similar properties to meditation but really means nothing more to me than to function by myself rather than interacting with others. Alone time isn't some new age millennial concept. We old guys used to spend a lot of time outdoors as kids sometimes with friends and sometimes without. I started running about three miles a day usually three days a week in junior high school. Before that I swam at the pool and rode my bike all over town. In those moments I was alone, inside my head devising plans and observing the world around me. That is what I consider alone time and I found it helps to break away from all that drags you towards stress. You still have to work and maintain your relationships but you could benefit from mindless distractions which can allow you to relax and consider new strategies as you learn the new ways of your second chance at life. I like to hike in the hills near my house, some people start fly-fishing.

I started writing this book for several and various reasons. This activity allows me to contemplate what I've experienced, gives me alone time, and a chance to share my ruminations with others. This adventure into the new and unknown is a way for me to explore new options and maybe even help someone else through a crazy chapter in their life. I believe that for you to write a book or just start a journal can be quite cathartic. Doing so also gives you an opportunity to share your view of your new life with your friends and family. Sometimes that share can help them understand where your head is at.

Probably the most important consideration about stress is the one passed on to me by my discharge doctor. You have just experienced one of if not <u>the</u> most stressful life-changing events in your life impacting you both emotionally and physically. Don't create more stress for yourself than you need to. Change your diet, start exercising more, destress, maybe quit drinking and/or smoking but focus first on the physical aspects of recovery from your event and prioritize future life changes based on what you think you can withstand. Above all remember, despite the sense of imperative you feel to become a new person you have spent many years as you were and it will take time, more time than you may believe. Not meeting your expectations is not failure but rather a chance to succeed later. Every day you wake up breathing is a gift and a new opportunity to achieve the satisfaction of being the person you believe you can be. Each night when you go to bed you came just a little closer didn't you?

4 DIET

Diet is a pretty important part of life to consider as you attempt to regain your health. I learned that if you don't eat you might die and nobody wants that right? For me it's hard to understand that many people start to or have already come to rely on medications and supplements to maintain their health and, let's be honest here, they still eat like crap. I despise medications and supplements simply because there are so many foods and spices that not only help but actually taste better than salt, fat, and sugar. Insert medical liability release here, These are my personal thoughts, not necessarily supported by medical professionals and is intended purely for consideration by intelligent persons. I don't wish for you to kill yourself by using my thoughts as your excuse to do stupid things! That being said I also realize that many people certainly and absolutely need to have medications, procedures, and such to continue breathing but some maybe not as much as they might think.

Anyway… The most surprising thing I learned is that I don't need to eat as much or as often as I thought I did before my event. Well, maybe I already knew that. More importantly I learned to consider my eating habits with more regard than I had to previously. If you're like me, in your younger days you could eat anything and everything and burn it off with little negative impact. Then you found that it would stick with you a little more each year. Seemingly suddenly you find yourself fat and slow. How did THAT happen, you think. Then boom, you have a heart attack and learn that all of the junk you've been eating has caused your body to wage an uprising!

The good news is that most of the damage to your body is reversible if you use logical consideration. For example you could just eat less and your body will react favorably and quickly, even if you still eat like crap. That doesn't mean you're doing what's best, just what's better. After my event I was literally afraid to eat anything that didn't fit the recommendations of medical staff. Can I drink coffee? No more bacon? No juicy steaks? What about fried foods? Guaranteed the doctors have given you plenty of medications to reduce the effects your past diet continues to have on your body. In fact I felt like that was the expectation, to continue with a poor diet and rely on the medications to reduce it's impact. But just in case you choose to eat better then you need to follow the low fat, low sugar, low salt, low carb path to longer life. Yuck!

Let's face it we probably gave up rabbit food as soon as we moved away from home. I did. Sweets are easier and tastier than fruit. Fried foods and crunchy foods are comfort foods used to help us alleviate stress and boredom as well as being convenient items at celebrations and gatherings. How many family functions do you go to where the salad maker is given the same warm welcome as the bringer of burgers? Exactly! I started by just not filling my plate three times and picking at stuff after eating at family get-togethers.

When I came home from the hospital I started out pretty good because I had just spent three days on my back eating hospital food portions and scared silly that I was going to die at any possible moment. Food was not a high priority! What food should I eat? The proposed menu given to me by the hospital was the ever severe; no salt, no fat unless it's, "healthy fat", no red meat, no cholesterol, and eat rabbit food menu with a solid focus on bird size portion control. Sure it might extend my life but at what expense? Remember George Burns telling his doctor that if he gave up cigars, whiskey, and women he saw no reason to want to live a longer life? I think we can identify with George! So what did I do? I tested my limits and experimented with different diet styles. Not strictly by any means, just that I went more for moderation rather than severe dietary item removal. Sorry, I still like my bacon, Porterhouse steak, and of course cheesecake. Just not six slices, two pounds, and half the cake respectively in one sitting.

Remember that my event was mitigated quickly enough to only cause muscle bruising I felt that I might have a bit more leeway than if I had incurred permanent damage. As I became stronger and began adapting to the effects of the beta blocker I started looking at dietary options that I could live with. There's the Mediterranean Diet, Ketogenic, Paleo, Atkins, and so many more. Each has stated benefits and each in it's own right might give you the healthy and enjoyable diet that will keep you breathing. I continue to attempt maintaining smaller portion controls and eating more rabbit food but it is a struggle because I do use food to try and relieve stress. This is a coping mechanism that I thought worked well in the past so I'm still adjusting away from that behavior. Try to be aware while you are eating in regards to how much of what and why. I found this to be the most effective management tool.

My greatest lesson about eating and therefore diet considerations is that I don't NEED nearly as much as I thought I did. Sure when I was seventeen I could eat everything in front of me and not show it but... I remembered that I didn't usually eat three squares a day and that one meal may have been the first all day and the last until tomorrow night. As I got older and living on my own eating even once a day wasn't a guarantee so yes, when food was in front of me, I ate like there was no tomorrow! Problem is that as I became a bit more mature, no, just responsible for someone besides myself, food became a more consistent thing. Now I had food around me all of the time and she could bake! I've always been skinny when single. Not so much when married and then there are the kids. All of the crap food that they like and is easy to make doesn't help. I was so used to scrounging their scraps because that food represented good money being thrown away, money that I had worked long and hard for. Just throw it away, because in your gut it's worse for you than in the trash can. Just imagine how much money you could save on groceries and eating out if you adjust your buying habits to your actual needs.

I believe that because in my youth, before my teens, I was unusually active and because I didn't have access to food all day long I was able to acquire great health. Don't get me wrong, I was skinny as a rail, but I could go all day, non-stop. Yes, I'm bragging but my point is that MY body had been accustomed to what is now referred to as, "intermittent fasting", something that stopped after I was married and somewhat stable. Anyone that knows me knows that, "stable", is always relative. I typically only eat at night, after work, and I try to only allow myself about an hour of feasting. If I minimize the high salt, high sugar, high junk stuff and eat well I can ride around at about two-hundred to two-hundred-fifteen pounds as of this writing. It has been close to two years since my event and I was admitted into the hospital at about two-hundred-fifty-six pounds. This was by no means a straight line progression but the trend still is less than more so I feel good about it and I can still eat lots of stuff that my cousin won't on her diet!

I believe another relevant consideration about what diet adjustment you make is your genetic background. I have to agree with the professionals on this but I think it goes deeper than genetic predisposition. I like to look at it as ancestry diet 101. Remember that your genetics go way past the last two, three, even four-hundred years. My background relative to my father is solidly Anglo-Saxon, Germanic, and then British primarily. My youngest daughter found out that our last name was associated with an area in Brittan. The significance of this side of my genetics and the consideration that on my mother's side of the chain includes Dutch descent as well shows that my ancestors were probably living near the coast, eating fish, wild game, and nuts and berries collected thought the year. This history might also explain my strong liver since beer was safer than water back then!

Using those considerations together with my personal experiences I came to develop a possible explanation for my genetic predisposition to heart disease and diabetes. Yes, I was also diagnosed with, "pre-diabetes" while in the hospital. Anyway; eating only when hungry, eating fresh meats, without salt and probably mostly fresh fish, splitting a loaf of bread with everyone, Eating rabbit food and the afore mentioned nuts and berries when available, and not having sugar would have determined I believe very specific results in how my body utilizes different food types and volumes. I also believe these considerations explain, to some extent, my compulsory cravings. Let's see what you think of these following examples.

If your body doesn't get a lot of what it needs it learns to stock-pile any amount of it and modify how it will process the item for greater benefit. For example, we all need salt but if we cannot receive what the body needs through a regular diet we begin to crave salty foods, especially when we're stressed for some reason. So in the salt example if the genetic brain says to hang on to any salt we get then the body will not shed the excess when there is any. If I'm close to being correct this predilection towards salt retention even when I consume large quantities consistently goes a long way towards explain how my blood pressure is elevated. By consistently cutting down my salt intake I've seen my blood pressure as low as 115/71. It still spikes at over 145/85 but compared to what my spikes were before the event. Look at the salt content in everything that comes from a package and compare. Check out dairy milk, WOW!

Now let's look at cholesterol. I considered the, "good fat",that everyone is hawking these days for better health. In my case my heart doctor told me that while my good fat numbers have gone up they have not and may not ever reach the standard levels. When I asked him why this was he suggested genetics. Hmm, genetics huh? What would cause my body to shed the good fats and retain the bad fats so effectively? Why would my body fight itself? I was listening to my body, giving it the things it craved. Not because it needed them but because it thought it did. What would cause that? So if the primary source of good fat for my ancestors was fresh fish and it was in good supply for multiple generations then genetics would adapt by shedding the excess quite efficiently because there would be more tomorrow. The bad fats on the other hand would be in short supply since wild game is lean and domestic livestock was not so abundant way back when.

By using this new to me hypothesis I believe that I now better understand what I'm fighting and therefore how to retrain my mind. That doesn't mean that I suddenly LOVE rabbit food! I just decided that my genetics are apparently accustomed to a NEVER ending supply of greens and my body doesn't retain the nutrients available for long. I realize that high fat meats were pretty, rare, see what I did there? There weren't large herds of cattle and a fat deer is a slow deer. This meant to me that I do need to scale back on the steaks and eat more chicken and fish. Relative to portion considerations I now eat half of a one-pound chicken breast most days instead of the one to two chicken breasts per meal I ate in my pre-event past. My bottom line on diet is, consider your biological and ancestral background, eat less, add new flavors and most of all if you are a dad and granddad like me, remember that your children/grandchildren share your genetic predispositions and they DO see your examples. Try to help them not experience what you did by showing them better, healthier behaviors and sharing your struggles with food. You are Superman to them but they are your whole world! To emphasize your responsibility to share your struggles with your family please consider that this is coming from someone who always plays the tough guy, even now, but by not sharing consider the struggles your family will face due to not knowing what you know today.

An additional consideration of my relationship between diet and heart health came to my attention recently which may help to explain some perplexing aspects of my health and apparent propensity for having heart issues. The excessive intake of sodium in my diet suddenly became a concern. I say suddenly because when I first came home I was salt and sugar scared. I read labels, changed cooking habits for my wife and myself, and started throwing away or not restocking, "bad", food items. All of this to the dismay of my wife! She loves salty and sugary foods and took these changes quite personally, and still does! So I recently started backing off from being the salt and sugar police and guess what. Suddenly my blood pressure is back to what it was before my heart attack!

According to the official medical diagnosis in my records my condition is described as Benign Hypertension. I never thought to question the heart doctor regarding this definition of hypertension and assumed that it was present but not contributing to my event? My recent raise in blood pressure caused me to reconsider that assumption. Now these considerations may or may not have been explained to me but I don't recall. After my event my blood pressure dropped immediately as did my resting pulse rate. I believed it was because of the beta-blocker, blood thinner, Statin, and daily aspirin regime. When the beta-blocker was eliminated from my routine I experienced a slight but temporary bump in heart rate and as my heart rate reduced my BP, blood pressure, stayed quite low. The results of dropping the blood thinner were similar and so I figured I had things well in hand. Until I was seeing my BP back to what it once had been.

After my event I was eating much more responsibly by eating less quantities and higher qualities. But suddenly I'm back to what I'd had. I had lost more than fifty pounds and I'm much more active than I have been since my late twenties. What was going on? Am I doomed to another heart attack or stroke or what? Most importantly, why was this happening?

Before I throw down my theory of why and what can be done I wish to present some information that I don't recall receiving at any time by any medical professional. Again, I iterate that I don't recall, not necessarily that I hadn't been informed. The information I recently learned was the impact that high BP can have on my kidneys! Short story is if you sustain high BP the blood vessels feeding your kidneys become damaged and that damage results in an ever diminishing capacity of the kidneys filtering effectively.

So back to the salt thing I presented earlier. Apparently salt or more accurately sodium attracts water. Excessive sodium seems to cause higher blood volumes and therefore higher BP which in turn causes systemic damage to the vessels and arteries and what have you. So guess what also has the capability of damaging your kidneys directly. Salt accumulations in your kidneys because they couldn't filter out excessive salt, sodium intakes before being inundated again!

The vicious circle that I just described is simply you ingest way too much sodium for long enough that you can't get rid of it. This in turn attracts water, which raises blood pressure, which injures blood vessels feeding the kidneys, which reduces their ability to remove sodium effectively, which causes your kidneys to retain sodium, which continues to build up. The total effect appears to end up as kidney failure which of course causes every other organ to quit! Scary shit huh? What scared me was learning that while some effects of long term excessive sodium intake can be reversed others cannot and actually could cause greater sensitivity and damage from sodium intake. This again puts us in a vicious cycle wherein we may indulge for a short term period and the kidneys react poorly. After that the kidneys become just that much more sensitive to your next indulgence. Can you see what I see? It looks terminal to me!

Back to me and my theory of why my BP suddenly increased and what I believe are contributing factors that increased my possible sodium sensitivity. Having been a skinny young guy I was more than a little vain about the waist size on my pants when I started getting fat. To put this change into perspective I am six foot, two and didn't get to two-hundred pounds until I was twenty-six years old. From then to the age of thirty-six I was about two-hundred-thirty to two-hundred-fifty pounds. My waist size went from a loose twenty-eight to a very snug thirty-six and up from there. I mentioned my vanity earlier to help you understand the possible correlation here. If I continually constricted my waist by wearing my pants too tight could I have constricted the blood flow to my kidneys? I wish to add that I had a runner's pulse up to the point that I first learned that my BP was elevated. Before that time my BP was considered marginally low. I understand that age and other factors including my family genetics play a part in it all but if obesity runs in the family, as it does mine, then I may also share with my family my vanity and practice of wearing constrictive pants.

My theory, which works in my head anyway, is that I have done things to myself in an unintentional and seemingly unassociated physical manner. I believe my behaviors are not an obvious consideration of the medical profession and are likely to be contributory to my circumstances. I think that possibly by wearing my pants too tight and holding them up with a belt pulled tight enough to cause my belly to literally hang over my waist I have inadvertently reduced blood flow to my kidneys. This reduction of blood flow would have been chronic and long term. Now let's get to the effects of sodium as presented previously. Sodium is in so many food items and at such high volumes that there is almost an absolute expectation of overwhelming the kidneys. Add to that the possible blood flow restriction to my kidneys which impedes their ability to function effectively. Now the kidneys are fighting a two sided battle, one that is essentially unbeatable since both can go on for a great length of time before the physical damage is apparent. But wait, when my BP was first observed as being elevated I was told it could be just a fluke or situational tension otherwise known now as white coat syndrome. When my high BP was observed consistently, about three years after the first abnormal observation, the answer wasn't salt but cholesterol.

To the best of my recollection I was counseled against high fats, red meats, high sugars, and excessive consumption. Salt was less of a consideration and certainly not given as much of a stated concern over cholesterol. The reference I was given regarding salt is that it would increase my blood pressure which would be hard on my vascular system, potentially causing another heart attack. Have you looked at the sodium content of your favorite foods? One example that totally took me by surprise was milk. I was raised like most people of my generation on two percent dairy milk. I like my milk. I used to drink about two gallons a week when I was a teenager and I was still consuming about half of our family's total weekly consumption, this with four kids trying to eat us out of house and home! After my heart attack I was advised that I may be sodium sensitive and should minimize my sodium intake whenever possible. Why would I look at milk? The milk I buy has one-hundred-thirty milligrams of sodium per one cup serving. A half-gallon container holds eight servings for a total of one-thousand-forty milligrams per container. I typically drank a half-gallon by myself in no more than three days just prior to my heart attack. Just in milk I was consuming at least three-hundred-forty-six milligrams of sodium per day.

Now add to that one item my excessive, "dad style", eating habits. Dad style is how I refer to making sure that no food goes to waste because of how hard I had to work to make the money to by the food. No way was I going to let that hard work go into the trash because of waste. Since my children all had moved out my darling wife has struggled to prepare appropriate amounts of food for two as opposed to six. She also doesn't like leftovers. So I'd eat leftovers on top of that day's dinner. Just look at the servings per container of any prepared food item and then multiply the sodium intake by at least three and you begin to see how much sodium was running through my system.

Current daily sodium intake recommendations are two-thousand milligrams per day, a teaspoon of salt. What is the solution? We already know the solution but if you're like me you didn't even know that there was a problem requiring a solution. I postulate that sodium intake is more of a contributing factor to my heart issues than possibly any other single consideration. I base my position on the many medical professionals I've consulted with since my heart attack. The primary cause of my event was that I had a rupture of an artery that released cholesterol. The release was caught in or near a heart valve and my blood immediately clotted around the cholesterol, blocking the artery completely. This situation was exacerbated by my higher blood pressures and the possibility of excessive Fibrin floating around in my blood looking for a hole to plug.

Getting older and living a less than subtle lifestyle helped bring about a more dramatic wake-up call than just consults with my family doctor would have accomplished. Having a heart attack was probably the most effective way that I could have been reached given my hard head! A thing that came to my attention when my blood pressure started to rise again was quite disturbing as well as a potential awakening in and of itself. Did you know that excessive sodium intake will severely affect your kidneys? Just pretend I haven't already been beating this horse for a second. Apparently there is a balance point between sodium and potassium that is the sweet spot of kidney function nirvana. Now it's one thing to upset that balance and yet probably quite another when you just slam your kidneys with vast amounts of one or both! Have you ever been suddenly buried under snow or sand and tried to dig your way out? Yeah that's about how I imagine my kidneys felt all of the time for probably forty plus years. No wonder they started slapping me around. Unfortunately I cannot hope to fully recover from that much abuse for so long. The results appear to be for me that not only do I need to diligently reduce overall consumption but to all but eliminate it to reduce further damage to my kidneys which seems to result in higher blood pressures immediately. The vicious circle is that each time I stress my kidneys I raise blood pressure which in turn more greatly stresses my kidneys. This causes less function capacity with every stress. The kidneys are somewhat resilient but they still lose a little every time. Consider now after more than forty years of ignorant blissful abuse that there has been some major damage that is irreparable.

If I have acquired any significant education about diet since my little event I believe the most important lesson is just because I use-ta-could doesn't mean that I was ever on the right track. Actually I have been very impressed that my body put up with me for as long as it did and as well as it did before finally grabbing me by the heart and shaking me up! Hard heads require hard lessons I guess. Within the first year of my heart attack I complained that I needed to become a chemist to develop a more appropriate diet intended to keep me alive a little longer. I still believe that but now I'm not complaining, I'm enthusiastic because I can explore new foods and spices that I've researched for health benefits. Together with my wife we have developed new to us meals and some meals that are very different from original recipes. I <u>almost</u> enjoy salads and I can <u>almost</u> stand beef liver. Always look at labels and then honestly consider your food portions when calculating. You could certainly attempt to claim ignorance when you go in for another heart attack but your claim will not save you from poor decisions, own yourself!

Water is necessary for life, but be careful how much you drink! I checked into what an average person should consume based on the latest daily quantities as recommended and learned that it is determined by your weight. In my case as of this moment that would be about 195 pounds. Per recommendations I should drink between 97.5 to 195 ounces of water per day. Let me tell you what I learned! The recommendations are supposed to take into account exercise or lack thereof. That is why the variance is so large. Even with that built-in tolerance I was peeing urgently and constantly!

Did I have an underlying issue? Prostate? Urinary? Something else? Nope! Here's what I learned and how I figured it out. The water recommendations do not take into account any water-like fluid, such as coffee. Everything I read informed me that coffee is a diuretic and therefore it would cause dehydration if anything. You may have realized while reading this book that I enjoy coffee and consider it a daily requirement! This means that I probably consume a substantial amount pretty much daily. I usually drink about 44 ounces a day. That is a very rough average as I drink a lot less some days and a lot more on other days. Per the accepted recommendations I did not include my coffee in my water intake measurements. If I drank 60 to 100 ounces of water a day plus my daily coffee intake I was urinating constantly and very urgently. Once I started to include my coffee consumption into the equation I found great relief! Consider all fluids in your daily water intake and watch how often you pee. Adjust according to your results. I think you might be, "relieved", to learn that your fine. If the results still concern you then, yes, you should visit your doctor and find out what's going on with you.

Sugar is not good for you. Heard that before right? Diabetics are insulin deficient and type 2 diabetics became insulin deficient. These were the statements that I grew up with and may still hold some weight. My experiences have been a reinforcement of currently suggested considerations. Maybe you're not insulin deficient but your body is insensitive to insulin because of how much it has to produce to keep up with incredible excesses of ingested sugar. Just like salt we usually consume so much more than our bodies can process. This is a statement recently supported by science. This is also a statement considered quite unfriendly to the food industry by the food industry.

Current guidelines are that an adult male should ingest 9 teaspoons or preferably less in a day. That equals 37.5 grams per day. Look at any processed food label and see what the serving size quantity of sugar is and then look at the serving size. Do the math! A twelve ounce can of soda has forty or more grams of sugar. One soda already puts me over the top! The reality as I see it is that we aren't insulin deficient but rather desensitized to insulin because our body is so overwhelmed with it and it has been shown to be at least as addictive as cocaine. Apparently the food industry and the government are very much aware of the problem with sugar and the connection to diabetes and overall organ health but… It was recently pointed out to me that daily recommended amounts of sugar are not stated on food labels. Don't believe me? Look for the percentage of daily recommended amounts for sugar on the next label you read. Not there is it? Maybe we need to put on our big boy pants and be more aware.

Personal observation of poor diet addiction especially relevant to sugar goes thusly. My ex-wife's mother and step-father were obese, diabetic, and one died of metastic pancreatic cancer and the other died shortly thereafter due to acute kidney failure. Short story is they were in terrible shape and died way too early with several factors present. They were good people and well loved by many but maintained a life-shortening lifestyle.

Both were very sedentary and both ate poorly. Part of the reason I'm not a huge fan of the medical community has to do with how they were advised and cared for in their location but more on that later. They were both heavier than I was before my heart attack. He had beat cancer and an earlier heart attack in his forties and they were both diagnosed as diabetic. They lived to eat, literally. They're favorite activity was to go to buffets and fill their plates several times. When they were home they sat in the living room in front of the tv until they went to bed. Exercise to them was to take their dog outside and wait for them to finish their business. Sounds pretty dangerous doesn't it?

When they were diagnosed with diabetes they were prescribed insulin injections, pretty common right? Well they figured out that if their blood sugar levels were too high that they could double and even triple their dosages to get it back down. They really thought they had a great solution and would eat even less responsibly than before. Guess what, that is not the answer. Their systems fought a losing battle until both finally lost and they both are now missing out on so much of what they wanted to experience with their grandchildren and great grandchildren.

Now on to the professional care they received in their last years. Doctors apparently did not advise them against abuse of their insulin since they always had enough. When she was in her final days at my daughter's home being treated by hospice we learned about the insulin abuse. They had been in rehabilitation/nursing homes on several occasions and we never heard about this abuse. His kidney function and diabetic condition while in a nursing home became so acute that his big toe turned black and had to be amputated. It gets better. After the amputation he ended up having another amputation of his calf. This secondary amputation has been attributed to the lack of timely care when the toe was treated. The infection had spread up his leg before the first amputation, apparently unobserved! When my youngest daughter and her best friend visited the nursing home and the doctor's office they learned that there was not a great deal of regard being given to the grandparent's health. Both have careers in social services, one in elder care and the other in child care. Let me tell you that things improved quickly and significantly after that visit!

Unfortunately the damage had been done and lives were unnecessarily shortened with terrible quality of life conditions due to the actions of, "professionals". The lessons that I learned and shared with my loved ones are the ones that I now share with you.

Self-advocate. My daughter's friend informed us that when the elderly lose their awareness the professionals seem to lose motivation to improve quality of life. Basically if you don't advocate for yourself then no one else will; even if they get paid to do so.

Try to change your lifestyle rather than rely on a chemical or procedural fix. There are reasons that you're in the shape you're in. even if you were ignorant to those reasons, once you know, you know. Step up buttercup!

Involve others in your health needs, especially as you become older. You may not have the information that others, even younger persons may know. At the very least when you are in a room with the doctor and someone that is concerned for your welfare the doctors tend to be a little more engaged…

Do your own research. Using the oldster in me I will refer to my primary research source as, "The Youtube". Sure there are some strange suggestions like drink your own urine but if you have a brain and look for real information that has been the quickest source of material for me. I do follow up with internet searches and the people I know and trust; and even a doctor or two.

Don't discount the value of psychological guidance. I say guidance because of my attitude about wholesale acceptance of anyonelse's professional opinion. If it sounds right and makes sense then great; But if it sounds like a way to keep getting your hard earned money then maybe not. We all be messed up in one way or another.

5 EXERCISE

Everyone LOVES exercise right? Yeah right, I know, but let's look at what exercise is today and what it once was, at least for me. When I was a kid I ran and rode bicycles and camped and hiked and and and so on. My point is that I stayed real active with little time to eat. I was too busy living not, "exercising". Later on I took up running. I ran about three miles a day about three days a week. I also took a clandestine trip to Virginia City from Sparks, Nevada by bicycle ONCE! I was a husband and father before my mom learned about my little adventure and the look she gave me then was still scary. In my late teens and early twenties I had limited access to food as a result of lifestyle choices and my financial capacity as a result of those choices.

You may ask what all of my bragging has to do with post event exercise considerations. I'm attempting to help you reframe what, "exercise", looks like to you. If you're a social animal and like to hang out at the gym, great! I don't need to drive miles away from home to spend hours working out on specialized machinery around people. I have a life, a family, and a job. I found myself in such a life threatening condition because I was too focused on what was going on around me and I was not concerned enough about what was going on inside of me. It was just easier to stare at the tv or web surf as I attempted to disconnect from the stresses and strains around me.

Since I was fairly active in my youth I had already built a strong cardio-pulmonary system which is probably the only reason I got as far as I did before my heart attack. I recently learned that my Southern cousin on my father's side had his first heart attack at the ripe old age of thirty-nine. I also believe that is why my body responded well to efforts to regain my physical health. Please take into consideration your personal physical history and the severity of damage done to your heart before diving into the deep end. I had blood thinners and beta blockers during most of the first year and they did greatly impact my strength and stamina. Take it easy and don't try training for a marathon right out of the gate!

One other reason that I prefer the great outdoors over the gym is fresh air. Have you been in a gym? I mean a real gym where everyone is working hard towards very high goals. Yeah they don't smell near as good as pine trees or sagebrush! I understand that you may not share my blessing of being in close proximity to some good hiking trails but even walking laps around your neighborhood will help you achieve some health benefits on a daily basis. Who knows, maybe your wife and kids could join you? That may be all that you can do for your health if you're really tore up but I know you will be surprised if you keep at it as to how effective a walk can be. I was mostly surprised at just how weak and unbalanced I had become over the many years of self-abuse. The pains <u>will</u> lessen and the distances will grow if you can keep going!

The information I looked at as I developed some kind of healthy activity patterns for myself is varied and depending on how gullible I might have been, can be very dangerous. As I said earlier I don't recommend training for a marathon. I recall being at a local park with my wife and observing a man walking laps around the park. The reasons why this guy caught my attention all came down to a very serious look of focus, an almost angry look that was matched by his pace. The gentleman looked like he'd been driven to make these hard laps but he didn't look like he was enjoying himself at all. His build was that of an old heavyweight boxer. You know, like he had been big and hard at one time but now he was just big? I nudged my wife and had her look his way. When she looked at him and then at me I said, "Must have had a heart attack". "Why?" she asked. "Because he don't look like he wants to be hot lapping the park, but more like he <u>has to</u>". You will be there my friend if you really want to get better and live longer. You will be pushing yourself wondering how you got so out of shape! Figure that out because you will need every motivation you can find to push past what you allowed to happen to your body and find a better way of living.

There are so many exercise and health regimes out there. Take a hard look at yourself, current condition and desired condition, and then look for suitable activities to reach your goals. Whenever you think things are too much for you at your age just look around at those your age doing more and looking better than you. My personal example has been Dwyane Johnson, he is my age, need I say more? Don't give yourself excuses; give yourself motivations to achieve more. Through a mindful diet and a relatively minimal exercise regime I have lost over sixty pounds. My exercise regime consists mainly of trying to get in about two and a half hours of walking per week with maybe an hour each week of arm focused weights. Not terrible right? I challenge you buttercup to figure out what you can do for you!

Something about exercise and subsequent medical testing of my condition I have to share with you because of my new understanding of how tests sometimes may not reflect reality. I currently possess a Commercial Driver's License and learned two years after my heart attack that there are some things that must be done to maintain the medical certification needed to keep my license. Things like I was supposed to have evaluation testing, both an examination by a cardiologist and an exercise treadmill test conducted within three months of my event. The Federal Motor Carrier Safety Administration, FMCSA, provide the medical requirements on their website. Even though on many occasions while I was in the hospital bucking for early release and afterwards during physical examinations I had mentioned the fact that I'm a CDL driver the cardiology practice did not seem to know what my needs were.

Point of fact, ignorance will not excuse you, so you need to diligently research any legal requirements you must fulfill because of your heart issues. I learned this and more when I went to get my D.O.T. physical done for my biannual medical recertification. After my event I learned that my medical certification will now be an annual requirement. The new to me requirements are that I must present to the doctor conducting the physical proof of a medical exam by a cardiologist within a year of the D.O.T. physical and documentation of a successful ETT which meets FMCSA standards. The ETT must be done every-other year. The way the D.O.T. recertification physicals are done meant that I suddenly learned that I had to have these things now and within three weeks of when I learned of the new requirements, new to me requirements. Talk about stress!

The challenges I suddenly faced required working within someone else's time frame both from the side of my license and the side of the medical practices and professionals. All I knew was that I had a short period of time to achieve these objectives without any personal control over when they could be accomplished. Needless to say I might have been a bit worked up and it showed in my blood pressure readings during all of my appointments and during my ETT. I learned how much I could force my blood pressure up by merely being emotionally tense and conversely I learned that I could exert emotional control and see some capacity to bring my BP down. I'm not great at it but I learned that I can and I'm sure you can too if you make the effort! The best example I can give is that when I arrived for the doctor's visit needed to set up the ETT my blood pressure upon arrival was 138/88. After believing that I had successfully achieved the necessary next steps to maintain my commercial license my BP was checked again. This time it was 102/68.

Regarding the ETT, I strongly suggest that you research the protocols and standards before the test. If I had I would have been more at ease during the test and with my results. In my test I achieved a MET value of 12.8. A MET is the estimated metabolic equivalents of a task. According to anything I can find regarding that number at my age I'm in pretty good shape! But the assessments stated by the medical staff that reviewed my results also showed that I have a, "Functional Aerobic Impairment of -8. According to what I can find that is not so good. What's going on I thought, so I looked into the protocols.

For example when I was given directions for test preparation I was told such things as to not eat a heavy meal before, I should wear comfortable clothes and shoes for running, and of course I should be well hydrated. My research, after the fact, advised that I should not have ingested alcohol, caffeine, or smoked cigarettes for at least three hours before the test. That would have been some handy information! I don't start my day without coffee and since the test took place at near noon I had smoked at least two cigarettes immediately before entering the office. May my ignorant behaviors have affected my results? Possibly. By the way, no I did not take a shot that morning!

In the exam room, according to my research, I should have been sat down quietly for a period to establish my resting stats. I was shuffled in, told to remove my shirt, chest razored and leads attached, and then my stats were taken. The actions taken by the staff administering this test were not necessarily in accordance with, shall we say best practices, and may have negatively impacted my test results.

Continuing down this path of observation, according to several sources I should have progressed to the final pace of 5.5 M.P.H at a 20% grade and then I should've been taken to a cool down pace before lying down to take my recovery stats. I was told that I'd be given the highest pace, work effort until I decided to end it. Yeah, no, none of that happened! The nurse ended the test and then told me that she would stop the treadmill in five, four, three, two, one, step on the rails. A five second cool down? Then immediately checking stats upright on the examination bed and wondering why my recovery wasn't instant!

In my opinion the culmination of all of these factors was that I went into the whole experience highly agitated and shall we say stressed but I still passed the exam sufficiently enough to maintain my commercial license. I decided to share this experience with you because I'm hoping you will be better prepared than I was and get more realistic information. Also I hope you sense my primary theme as I write this book; Research and self-advocate! Do not _ever_ totally rely on the guidance of the medical community! It's your life, not theirs; you have much more to lose than they do if you don't care for yourself as you need to. I have seen too many people live shorter and less than optimum lives because they allowed the medical professionals being paid to _serve_ their patients treat them with less than respect.

6 SLEEP

Ahh sleep, wonderful elusive sleep. Do you know what I'm talking about? I'm pretty sure you do. Before my heart attack I usually went on five or less hours of sleep daily. I just went until I couldn't. This had served me well when my work and family demanded it and of course I'm tough, there's no reason to think I can't be that way forever. Right? Yeah, wrong. We all need sleep just like everyone says and none of us are immune to that need.

Now how much sleep an adult needs in a given timeframe is still up for discussion in my estimation but here are some things I've looked at and have found to be helpful to me, anyway. First is consideration of you physical and emotional stresses in a day. If you aren't very physical but are wound up all day your body is just as spent as if you worked a shovel. You know the one with a metal pointy end and a long wooden handle? Physical labor does benefit the body in balanced amounts. Non-physical, mindful stress benefits nothing but it causes chemical reactions within your body that hurt way worse than physical fatigue.

In my efforts to relearn how to operate this machine of mine I have explored many diverse disciplines. When I say explore please understand that I haven't sought medical, religious, or even the experiences of others that have had heart attacks directly. Rather I have conducted informal research on the internet, especially on the Youtube site, considered my personal experiences and the experiences of those I watched before and after their heart attacks. Oh yes and don't forget the physiological aspects of sub-atomic Quarks! All in all my cogitations come down to we probably could sleep better and longer to achieve greater health.

A Yogi I found on Youtube, Sadhguru, essentially stated that if you can find rest in your mind you will not require as much sleep. I have interpreted Sadhguru's perspective to be that if you are more at rest then your mind and body require less of the recuperative benefits of actual sleep. His logic is sound in my opinion and I do strive for that restful state of being but I believe it will take extensive time and practice for me to find that place!

Circadian Rhythm is expressed as the very specific genetically and environmentally optimal times for sleeping. The rhythm is based on light and dark as well as temperature and meal times. This consideration seems to state that you have to operate in the very specific period of the day without more than a two hour variation in either direction to receive optimal benefits. Hmm, So I usually get up around seven AM and try to get to bed by eleven PM during the week. On Friday night I struggle to go to bed before one AM and if I fail in that struggle I will be up as late as four AM. So on the weekends if left to my own devices I usually sleep in to around ten or eleven AM. When I wake late on the weekends I actually feel better than if I sleep on my weekday schedule. So which is out of whack? My natural sleep rhythm, or the Circadian Rhythm?

My youngest son bought me a Fitbit Blaze when I was attempting to escape the hospital. I tell you this to give credence to statements about my sleep patterns. For instance I learned that I spend the majority of my sleep time in what is referred to as light sleep. If I'm fortunate I will get around an hour each night of deep sleep. I also usually have a total of around another hour of being awake each night. This is typical regardless of what day of the week or what time I go to sleep. I've also found almost no correlation between sleep stages and heart rate.

Basically I haven't found that perfect sleep period or sleep state from which to help me manage my heart rate or blood pressure, at least through direct awareness. Instead I found that being calm and relaxed before attempting to sleep is, and logically so, the best way to get the best rest. The standard recommendations of evening meditation and white noise can help but it's more about you finding your best headspace. It all comes down to what you do in your mind. If you decide to stress or worry on something then nothing external will help you rest. Sure there are sleeping pills but then that's not really rest is it? You have to decide that whatever is troubling you in the moment is not so important in that particular moment. It will take practice and becomes a new skill. I say a new skill because if you're like me, allowing any troubling thought to impede sleep is already a well-developed skill that you will have to unlearn. Running until complete exhaustion is no longer doable.

The best sleep advice that I can pass on from my experiences thus far is that if you've had an event yourself then you must realize that you ain't the man or woman you used to be! Our bodies can be so rude when they've finally had enough abuse. The abuses of insufficient sleep have considerable impact on your overall health. You <u>need</u> to take a breath, and then remember to take care of yourself first.

Everyone around you that truly cares will be stepping in and up to help you. Sometimes without your consent! My children and their spouses came at me and gave me my first <u>intervention</u> immediately after I was out of the hospital. They in no uncertain terms made me understand the way I would be expected to behave by relying on them to help me with the more strenuous tasks that I have. Their concern was sweet as hell but also quite maddening. First because I was now being talked to like I've talked to them since they were children and second because I knew they were right. I didn't accept that they were right but I knew they were right. Let go for a little bit and then take on what you can. If it's too much now, back off and try again later. Get your rest whenever the mood strikes and use everyone's concern for your wellbeing for as long as they'll let you!

7 SMOKING TOBACCO

Smoking, the Devil incarnate according to every pundit today. Smoking seems to be solely responsible for so many ailments. I was told that it was a major contributing factor to my cataracts! I couldn't have possibly damaged my eyes back in my twenties when I arc burned them on several occasions while welding. My cataracts were essentially blamed solely on my smoking and other bad habits until I met with my eye surgeon. He informed me that lifestyle and diet seem to have very little to do with a person's propensity to acquire cataracts. Cataracts like most things seem to be of a genetic origin.

If you're from my generation, you know, generation X, then you likely grew up with many people smoking in cars, restaurants, grocery stores and the like. Yes, even around children in enclosed spaces. As I was told in my younger days it was a good thing I started smoking and drinking coffee at such a young age because it stunted my growth and kept me under seven foot tall! Smoking wasn't evil but rather just a thing that some did and others didn't. We all grew up different and some smoked and quit and others still smoke. I still smoke although certainly not as much as I did before my event. As it was explained to me by a medical professional I lean on smoking as a way to deal with all kinds of circumstances and have done so with what became the longest known companion I've had. My relationship with smoking is much like an old friend that I've hung out with for close to forty years. I have few acquaintances and even fewer people that I call friends with whom I've held such a long relationship! That isn't a relationship so quickly dismissed, at least not by me.

Smoking is included in the many behaviors and predilections of those like me who have had or could likely have atherosclerosis. Smoking is considered one of several indicators of a person's likelihood of possessing the physical attributes responsible for having a heart or stroke issue. Recently I came across a somewhat contrarian consideration; What if these behaviors were not the contributing factors of heart disease but rather shared behaviors, only indicators but not necessarily contributing factors?

I'm not saying that's the case but there is a bit of consideration out there that a person with the genetic predispositions for heart disease also, typically, have the same likelihood to drink alcohol to excess, smoke cigarettes, overeat, and function in high stress environments. All of these and the inclusion of poor quality sleep and diet make a great recipe for disaster. Is it the behaviors or the attraction of the behaviors due to genetics? Nature or nurture or all of the above? I don't know but thirty years ago heart disease seemed to be a secret and silent killer with no apparent connection to any of these behaviors.

So we all can agree that smoking is bad for us physically. The research out there is overwhelmingly abundant showing proof of the harms from smoking. The emotional attachment to smoking like the comparison made by the doctor as and old and reliable friendship is quite accurate in my case. I feel the need to keep up the relationship but I continue to work towards more distance from my old friend and learning to handle things without that support. I'm not done and I'm not always sure that I will completely walk away but I want to be around and harassing the general public for as long as I find value in doing it!

Fortunately every time I resist having a cigarette I give my body a longer recovery period from the last one. I also gain breath and strength which allows me to do more. Another benefit of slowing down and hopefully ending the relationship is substantially reduced overall body pain. Unfortunately I cannot offer a sure cure since I haven't found one that works for me but any reduction is an improvement. One caution I will throw out there is regarding cessation drugs. Smoking is unhealthy and is an aspect of your personality that can be modified but some of those drugs will actually turn you into a different person. Some people that I've spoken with in the past have told me that what they became as a result of the side effects was not necessarily pleasant. Try to find a way to end the relationship well and on your terms. Maybe a dinner and a movie with some flowers?

8 DRINKING

The relationship I have with smoking is much like the one I have with Jack, you know Jack. Jack will still party with me and help enhance the joy of just about any activity but like any good friend he lets me know when I've gone too far. He usually does it with a gentle nudge at first but if I ignore his guidance I pay for it! If you know Jack then you've been there and learned accordingly, maybe. I know many that are in substantially worse shape than me still don't get the hint. My point is that I grew up around drinking and usually to excess. I observed it as a child and even then I partook on many occasions. I also used my youthful experiences to hone some fairly exceptional skills in the art of consumption. Many of us have, and some still do.

When the discharging doctor stopped by to give me and my wife guidance on how to behave at home she looked me in the eye and said, "The days of two gallons of whiskey a night are gone." I responded with, "Those days had been long gone for a while." Apparently I looked like a lush? Anyway, since alcohol is a consumption item it probably should have been included in the diet section but since drinking is more so an activity with no connection to nourishment of the body whatsoever I felt it needed it's own chapter.

The science is pretty simple; Alcohol is caused by sugars being fermented with yeast. When alcohol is consumed at any level inside our body it has to be processed and filtered by our organs. You've heard of psoriasis of the liver? Too much alcohol overwhelms the liver and it basically dies inside of you. Everything is taxed by excessive consumption. Your kidneys, heart, and brain are especially and extraordinarily stressed by too much booze. I know of at least one person that recently experienced a stroke in his sleep after his average night at the bar. I say an average night for _him_ as he typically was and probably still is at the bar more nights than not. He was fifty-four when he experienced his first _known_ stroke. The stroke was enough to affect his facial muscles and some motor skills. Fortunately he didn't experience a more intense stroke and he was able to go to work where he was ordered by his daughter to get checked out by a doctor!

Strokes and heart disease seem to go hand in hand. If you're likely to have one you may have the other as well. The lifestyle indicators are also typically the same. You likely smoke, allow considerable stress to affect your psyche, take crazy risks, eat too much of the unhealthy stuff, live on little, if any sleep, and generally let yourself be a crash test dummy. I've stated in other parts of this book that our risk indicators have typically been stated as the causes of our health issues but I'm kinda leaning toward consideration that the indicators are just that, indicators. People with these predispositions and outlets are likely to drive themselves into dangerous and life-shortening physical and emotional conditions as a result of personal temperament.

Less is better and none would probably be best. If abstinence is unlikely then like with all other potentially life-shortening activities and decisions there will be consequences. When or how these consequences manifest themselves will not be on your terms and will certainly cause you and yours pain and suffering.

9 GOING FORWARD

Here we are, near the end of my rants and raves. I know that I feel better, don't you? I have a family that I love deeply and feel quite blessed at having them in my life! I worked harder to improve my health after my event than I might have because of them. I know that not everyone has these blessings and motivations in their lives to help. If you find yourself without motivation you will likely find great difficulty attempting to extend and enhance your life through the tough choices you have ahead of you. Please find something or someone!

This chapter is my summary of what I've learned and what could help you. You may learn from these words if you've experienced the, "event", or if someone you care about has and you're looking for ideas to help. You may just want to understand what they could be dealing with if you're a concerned bystander. If you've been diagnosed with a cardiovascular health problem then I hope you're reading this to find out what others have done to improve their circumstances.

The bullet list of things to do going forward:
- Celebrate! You survived to live another day!
- Annoy your loved ones with lots of affection!
- Annoy your loved ones with your attempts at self sufficiency
- Let others help
- Conduct your own research on everything
- Rest more
- Eat less
- Eat better
- Take time for yourself. Whether that is exercise, meditation, or hobbies
- Smoke less if at all
- Drink less if at all
- Reflect on where you find yourself and where you'd like to be
- Share your experience with loved ones because they got scared too!
- Live and love like you're on borrowed time because now you know that all of our time on this planet is and was borrowed!

The bullet list of things to not do going forward:
- Don't resent yourself for past actions. You now have another chance to do better.
- Don't be afraid to live. That would suck!
- Don't continue to use past stress reduction behaviors because they brought you to the brink.
- Don't just accept things as they're described or prescribed, if you know what I mean.
- Don't give up when you fall short of your objectives. Learn from the mistakes and try again.
- Don't go commando!, Opps, wrong list!
- Don't go Superman stupid. Living on the edge put you here, pull up dude!

I purposely presented more do's than don'ts. Where you focus your energies, negative or positive can have tremendous consequences. Everybody tells us to find our, "happy place". Create your happy place where you're at buddy. I'm not recommending that you quit your present life but rather that you clarify in your mind what your real happiness is really all about.

Sure the big car, big house, big whatever is better than the smaller version but is it worth killing yourself to acquire? If you make changes based on your health and true needs I believe you will be happier. I'm not saying don't try stuff that could cause unneeded stress. I am saying that you are alive and that could give you another chance to live a life you want!

AFTERWORD

My position as I've offered here is that we are omnivores. We are omnivores in dietary consumption obviously but also in experiences. Many of us that have experienced a heart attack knowingly pursued high risk lifestyles for so many reasons. Regardless of the presumption of positive or negative framing of the decisions we've made we made them and the results were not so good. I grew up with the mantra of try, try again. I then applied that attitude to some pretty positive efforts but I also did the same when it came to smoking, drinking, and life-threatening stunts. Maybe that's how we all are and maybe not.

I started writing this book because I wanted to keep track of what I'd learned since my event. I soon considered this effort as a great passive-aggressive way to share my side of this experience with my family and friends. In the end I figured that I could achieve all of his and maybe more. What if I could loser the learning curve for those just coming from where I was? What if I could give first hand understanding to those that have seen a loved one go through a heart attack? How about the ones that just learned from their doctor that they're at considerable risk of suffering from cardiovascular impairments? Being the altruistic being that I am, ha ha, I truly hope that this book does all of that and maybe more.

Please live your life with meaning and love because as they say work and things only have value if you enjoy yourself. I have enjoyed my experience putting these words on to paper so to speak. I also very much enjoy living near the edge but I figure maybe I could get a little further from it and have more precious time to live, love, and just observe what is. Thank you for deciding to walk with me as I've shared and I hope you have many great days ahead of you!

ABOUT THE AUTHOR

David Seabolt lives in Northern Nevada and was blind-sided by a heart attack shortly after his fiftieth birthday.

www.ingramcontent.com/pod-product-compliance
Lightning Source LLC
Chambersburg PA
CBHW050343290526
45785CB00006B/2618